THE GLUCOSE UPSET:

LIFE-ALTERING ABILITY TO CONTROL BLOOD SUGAR

By

Victor T. Rice

Copyright© by Victor T. Rice 2023. All right reserved

TABLE OF CONTENTS

INTRODUCTION

Our favorite theory postulates that desire behaviors and associated brain changes may sustain very alluring meals with lots of added sugar. Well-thought-out therapies and mechanistic studies are needed to explore this fascinating idea thoroughly. Notwithstanding the possibility that the brain's reward system and the "addictive" quality of tasty foods contribute to the high daily intake of added sugars among Americans, the prevalence of added sugars in today's diet and the powerful advertising of the food industry may also have a significant impact.

Based on the research, the majority of Americans eat more added sugar than is recommended for optimal health. This studies provide support for the existing recommendations to reduce added sugar intake in US diets, as do the effects of much other research.
In order to lower the global daily sugar intake to 25 grams, the World

THE GLUCOSE UPSET

Health Organization released recommendations earlier this year. An expert-led "wake-up call to rethink our diet" has also prompted the UK government to halve the recommended daily sugar consumption. Our only option is to decrease because we are in a bind with sugar. There is nothing wrong with it, provided we are aware of the initial quantity of sugary food we are ingesting.

Not all of the time is reality this simple. Reducing sugar may seem complicated and perplexing since nutrition labels sometimes need to be clarified, and there is a widespread lack of knowledge about sugar guidelines. You may be surprised even if you think you're eating a healthy amount because it doesn't even account for the hidden sugar that may be present in certain unexpected everyday meals, that we consume much too much sugar, far too often, is the one thing we do know about it. However, how much sugar is too much? Where does it originate,
why is it even bad for us, and have we always eaten this much beforehand? After hearing the word "glucose," what comes to mind?

Do you struggle and want to ignore it? Can you think of anyone else who should be worried besides those with diabetes? Does this lead you to believe that glucose is harmful emotionally? For what purpose does glucose serve?

Should you encounter any of the above-described responses, keep calm you are not alone. It's more complicated to understand what glucose really does in your body,

though. We need glucose to survive, despite the myth surrounding it—glucose is the sugar that our bodies need as fuel—which often depicts it as the villain in every diet. To thrive correctly, we even need it.

You may need to include extra glucose (also known as carbs) in your diet.

CHAPTER 1

Understanding what Glucose is all about

Your body converts the sugar known as glucose, which it gets from the food that you eat, into glucose, which it then utilizes as a source of energy. The word glucose is derived from the Greek word that means "sweet," and it is a form of sugar.

If you have high glucose levels in your blood, it can have an effect on your kidneys, eyes, and other organs over time. Glucose enters the body's cells from circulation so that it may be stored and utilized as a fuel source. Glucose entering the cells of the body from the circulation.

Patients who have diabetes have blood glucose levels that are much higher than typical. Either the cells in their bodies do not respond to insulin as well as they should, or their bodies do not have enough insulin in their systems.

Glucose Is Not Your Competitor.

Glucose is essential for human life despite the fact that some persons are more hypersensitive to its effects than others. Think about using some basic ways to make your body more sensitive to glucose, such as ingesting one tablespoon of apple cider vinegar mixed in water before

each meal or giving veggies more importance than protein and fat when you are eating carbs. It's possible that making these minor alterations will have a large and beneficial effect on your mood, level of energy, and mental clarity.

Certain people likely require healthier carbs in order to keep their hormones in check, maintain emotional equilibrium, and maintain consistent amounts of energy. If you find that following a low-carb diet is making you feel unwell, you might want to experiment with adding a small amount of complex carbs to your diet to see if this provides you with more energy.

Why Is It Significant to Have Glucose?

All of the cells in the human body require energy in order to carry out their functions. It is in charge of carrying out the metabolic tasks that are essential to our continued

existence. The glucose in your bloodstream provides fuel for your muscles, brain, and a variety of other organs and tissues throughout your body.

In addition to this, it is present in larger structural molecules such as glycolipids and glycoproteins. The human body precisely controls the amounts of these substances. The results of having levels that are abnormally high or low might be catastrophic. However, it does have inevitable consequences that could be fatal.

• It provides a source of mental fuel

Glucose supplies the brain with around 80 percent of the energy it requires on a daily basis. Due to the fact that our brain is unable to retain glucose and has a high need for power, glucose must always be accessible. Hypoglycemia, also known as a quick drop in blood sugar, can be prevented thanks to the many defense systems that are present in the human body. Because of this, one's cognitive abilities might start to deteriorate. Headache, lightheadedness, disorientation, loss of focus, anxiety, irritability, restlessness, slurred speech, and decreased coordination are some of the most common symptoms of hypoglycemia that can occur in the brain.

Seizures and coma are possible side effects of a large decrease in blood sugar.

• Increasing the Fuel for the Muscles

Skeletal muscles typically make up between 30 and 40 percent of total body weight. This varies depending on factors such as your age, gender, and current level of physical fitness. The reading activity stimulates the skeletal muscles to consume a considerable quantity of glucose, which has the desired effect. In contrast to the brain, the skeletal muscles store glucose as glycogen, which, during exercise, is rapidly broken down into glucose. The brain, on the other hand, keeps blood sugar as glucose.

•Provides the organs and tissues with the necessary energy for them to carry out their functions.

The human body is comprised of a wide array of organs and tissues, each of which is capable of extracting energy from its own unique combination of fuels. Glucose is either the major or the only source of energy for many of

the essential tissues and organs in the body, such as the brain and the skeletal muscles. Other tissues and organs include the red and white blood cells, as well as the cornea, lens, and retina of the eye in the eye. Other tissues and organs include the digestive tract. The many organs and tissues each contain a variety of additional components.

Glutamine is the principal source of fuel for the cells that are found in the small intestine, despite the fact that these cells also take up glucose from the food that is consumed and transport it throughout the body. Because of this, it is now feasible for a greater quantity of glucose to enter the organs and tissues that are dependent on sugar.

How Does Your Body Handle the Task of Managing the Production of Glucose?

The most common sources of it are foods that are high in carbohydrates, such as bread, potatoes, and fruit. As you chew and swallow, food travels down your pharynx and into your stomach. It is broken down into very little fragments by the enzymes and acids in that environment.

During this procedure, glucose is released into the bloodstream.

After traveling through your digestive tract, it reaches your bloodstream, where it is absorbed. Following that, it is absorbed by your circulation. Once glucose is circulating in your bloodstream, insulin assists your cells in taking it up.

Energy Storage Available

Your body's job is to make sure that the concentration of glucose in your blood stays the same at all times. Beta cells in your pancreas do a glucose level check on your blood at regular intervals of a few seconds each. When we eat, our beta cells respond by secreting insulin into the bloodstream, which causes our blood glucose levels to rise. The absorption of glucose by muscle cells, fat cells, and hepatocytes is significantly aided by insulin's presence.

As a source of energy, the bulk of the cells in your body are fueled by lipids, carbohydrates, and amino acids, which are the fundamental components of proteins. Regardless of this, it acts as the principal source of energy for your brain. For information to be processed, nerve cells and chemical messengers both need to be present. Without it, the functions of your brain would be severely compromised.

After your body has used up all of its available energy, the glucose that is left over is stored in your muscles and liver in the form of little bundles known as glycogen.

Your body has the capability of storing energy for as long as a day at a time.

Your blood sugar levels will naturally drop after you have abstained from food for a few hours. Your pancreas is no longer producing insulin because you have diabetes. The pancreatic alpha cells are the ones that initiate the production of the one-of-a-kind hormone glucagon. It instructs the liver to begin the process of releasing glycogen from storage and converting it back into glucose.

This enters your system and replaces your stockpiles so that you may continue to function well until you have another opportunity to eat. In addition, your liver can generate glucose by breaking down lipids, amino acids, and other waste products.

Can Glucose Substances Be Produced By Plants?

Their leaves are the first parts of the plant to absorb moisture and carbon dioxide from the surrounding air and soil. Water undergoes oxidation within the cells of plants, which also results in the reduction of carbon dioxide and the accumulation of electrons. During this process, water is turned into oxygen, while carbon dioxide is transformed into glucose. While the oxygen is discharged into the atmosphere, it is the glucose molecules that are responsible for storing the available energy.

Plants require this energy in order to mature, continue their growth, and make more molecules, such as cellulose and starch. Plants cannot survive without cellulose for the construction of their cell walls, yet the portions of plants and their seeds store starch for use as a food source. Some foods, including rice and wheat, contain a significant

amount of the nutrient starch. In its most basic form, photosynthesis may be described as a complicated series of chemical reactions that results in the production of glucose, a fundamental sugar from the gases carbon dioxide, water, and oxygen, with the aid of light.
On the other hand, not all forms of photosynthesis are created equal. The majority of plant species produce a molecule with three carbon atoms that are called 3-phosphoglyceric acid when they eat carbon (C3).

Eventually, glucose will be released by this molecule. The resources that are present in a plant's environment are what decide whether or not it will develop photosynthesis. C4 photosynthesis, for instance, helps plants develop even in conditions when there is little light and water by increasing carbon content.

CHAPTERS TWO

The Importance Of The Glucose Spike And The Causes

There are a number of books and articles on diets that claim that they can treat and prevent type 2 diabetes as well as rises in blood glucose. But what exactly are spikes in blood glucose, and why is it essential to keep them under control? Without a doubt, our bodies monitor the amounts of glucose that are present in our blood.

A blood sugar spike occurs after eating whenever there is an excessive rise in the levels of glucose in the blood. Blood sugar levels are generally well-managed, but factors such as diet and lifestyle can hamper the body's capacity to do so, particularly as people become older and gain weight. This is especially true when people gain weight. When glucose levels in the blood remain elevated for an extended period, a condition known as prediabetes can develop. If this condition is not addressed, it can progress to **type 2 diabetes.** The number of people who are diagnosed with type 2 diabetes has grown by a factor of 10 during the past four decades. People are increasingly being diagnosed with diabetes at younger and younger ages.

In both the United Kingdom and the United States, prediabetes affects almost one-third of the population, although only one in ten people are aware that they have the condition. It is a significant issue that is only going to become worse in the future.

Why Are Blood Sugar Spikes So Dangerous?

The arteries become damaged over time when there is a high quantity of sugar in the circulation. This can lead to consequences such as heart disease, renal disease, and diabetic eye disease in the affected individual. It is of the utmost importance to determine whether or not you have high blood sugar in order to get it under control and reduce the likelihood of causing harm to your body.

Can I Get My Blood Glucose Levels Checked for Spikes?

An accurate determination of whether or not your blood glucose levels are persistently high can only be made via the use of a blood test. A certified medical expert, such as your primary care physician, should do this test, which is known as the HbA1c test. If you have diabetes, you should have this test done on a regular basis. Make advantage of the Diabetes UK self-assessment tool in order to determine whether or not you are at risk of acquiring type 2 diabetes.

What exactly is a test for HbA1c?

The formation of glycated hemoglobin, also known as HbA1c, takes place when glucose, or sugar, in the blood binds to red blood cells. Due to the fact that your body is unable to utilize glucose effectively, an increased amount of it adheres to blood cells and accumulates, which can be harmful. The range that is considered normal is from 26 to 41 mmol/mol. You put yourself at risk of getting type 2 diabetes if your blood sugar levels grow above specified thresholds. Type 2 diabetes may be reversible with early diagnosis and aggressive treatment.

What Can I Do To Control My Blood Glucose spike Levels And Decrease My Risk Of Type 2 Diabetes?

• If you have spikes in your blood sugar, the most important thing you can do is avoid meals that include a lot of processed carbohydrates, such sugar and white flour (also known as "white carbs"). Your diet might benefit from more fruit, vegetables, and healthy grains. In place of sugary drinks, try drinking sugar-free coffee, sugar-free tea, water, or plain milk.

*Adhere to a dietary regimen that is rich in "nutritious fats and oils," such as those abundantly present in various nuts, seeds, avocados, and olive oil.

• Include vegetables and pulses like chickpeas, beans, and lentils in your diet as part of high-fiber carbohydrate meals.

• To meet your daily protein needs, consume whole foods such as eggs, fish, chicken, and turkey; unsalted nuts, seeds, and lentils are all good options.

THE GLUCOSE UPSET

• You should engage in more physically taxing activities. Problems with maintaining normal blood glucose levels are frequently brought on by seventies. If you don't work your muscles frequently enough, fat will accumulate inside the fibers, insulin resistance will develop, and your blood glucose levels will rise.

Becoming more physically active is the quickest and most straightforward approach to change this. Walking is an effective method for managing blood sugar levels. Less than 5,000 steps are covered by the typical person on a daily basis. The optimal number of steps to walk each day is 10,000, and you should endeavor to do that. Make an effort to proceed carefully initially.

Keep a record of the meals you eat.

While you are eating, you need to pay attention. Some people choose to forego eating breakfast in favor of consuming two more substantial meals later in the day: lunch and dinner. This may induce a surge in your blood sugar. Consume a number of well-balanced meals in addition to a couple of snacks during the day. It is best to have several smaller meals rather than one or two really large ones.

You also have the option of separating your food into two distinct meals for the day. At five o'clock, eat the first part of your meal. Instead of having one at seven o'clock and the other half a few hours later, we'll have both at once.

The Reason Behind Working Out

The usage of insulin can be improved with exercise, which in turn helps with glucose control. After you have finished eating, there is absolutely no reason for you to sit down on the couch. After supper, going for a short stroll may assist in preventing sharp increases in blood sugar levels. When you exercise, your muscles demand more blood flow than expected, which means that the amount of glucose that your intestines have to digest is reduced.

Foods That Cause An Increase In The Level Of Blood Sugar

A lot of individuals are under the impression that foods high in sugar are mostly to blame for when their blood sugar levels surge. They are nevertheless obtainable through the consumption of foods like white bread and potatoes.

On the other side, eating processed meals, drinking sugary drinks, and consuming refined grains will generally, adhere to a dietary regimen that is rich in "nutritious fats and oils," such as those abundantly present in various nuts, seeds, avocados, and olive oil. glycemic index of dextrose is 100, and it is a form of glucose that may be derived from grain sources like wheat or corn. It is commonly present in sweets, which can lead to an increase in one's blood sugar level.

The following is a list of meals that will increase your blood sugar level:
• Goods prepared in the oven • Foods prepared in the fryer
• Mashed potatoes • Pizza
• Cereals for breakfast that are high in sugar
• Bread made with whole grains

Foods For Healthy Blood Sugar Control
If you absolutely must consume meals with a high glycemic index, combine them with items that have a low glycemic index in order to slow digestion and maintain a healthy glucose level.

Meals that have been processed take longer to digest than whole meals. Take the lowly apple, for example. Although apples naturally contain fructose, often known as fruit sugar, their glycemic index is lower than that of other fruits because the fiber in apples is more challenging to digest, which in turn restricts the amount of glucose that is released. On the other hand, apple juice will induce a far more rapid rise in blood sugar due to the processing of fruit juices, which eliminates part of the fiber from the fruit.

Emphasize foods that are high in fiber, such as brown rice, beans, and whole grains. In addition, your body takes a more extended amount of time to digest meals that are hard, cold, or unripe. For instance, eating unripe bananas will not have the same effect on your blood sugar levels as eating mature bananas.

The following are some meal options that might help you sustain appropriate blood sugar levels:
Apples, Almonds, cashews, and walnuts • Black beans, kidney beans, and pinto beans • Broccoli • Cauliflower •Chickpeas • Dark chocolate • Full-fat dairy • Oats

Diseases Related To Glucose Content In The Blood, Such as Diabetes

The usual response of your blood sugar level after eating is an increase. After a few hours, it begins to drop as insulin begins to transfer glucose into the cells of your body. Your blood sugar levels should be below 100 milligrams per deciliter (mg/dl) in the three to four hours between meals. This number is known as your blood sugar level when you haven't eaten anything.

Diabetes is an illness that occurs when a person has an abnormally high quantity of sugar (glucose) in their blood. Diabetes is also known as sugar diabetes. Diabetes results from your body's inability to create an adequate amount of insulin. In the absence of insulin, your body will not be able to extract the required amount of energy from the food you eat. In a healthy body, the pancreas secretes the hormone insulin is in charge of transferring blood sugar into cells. Diabetes is characterized by either an insufficient production of insulin by the pancreas or an insulin response that is impaired in some way.

There exist some distinctions between type 1 and type 2 diabetes.

• The insufficient production of insulin by the body is the hallmark of type 1 diabetes. This causes the immune system to attack and kill pancreatic cells that produce insulin.

A person with type 2 diabetes' cells are incapable of absorbing insulin. Thus, the pancreas must produce more insulin in order for cells to absorb glucose. Gradually, the pancreas will sustain damage that will impair its ability to generate enough insulin to meet the body's needs.

It is impossible for glucose to enter cells if there is not enough insulin. There is still a fair amount of glucose in the blood.A patient may develop hyperglycemia if their blood glucose levels are over 200 mg/dl 125 mg/dl or two hours following a meal after a fast.

Because your arteries are the blood vessels that provide oxygen-rich blood to your organs, an overabundance of glucose in your body might harm them. Having elevated blood sugar raises your risk of contracting any of the following specific diseases:

• Heart disease, heart attack and stroke risks/probabilities

Neurological trauma; renal disorders;
A disorder that affects the eyes is called retinopathy.
Diabetic patients should routinely check their blood sugar levels. You may help keep blood glucose levels in a healthy range and prevent problems like these by exercising frequently, maintaining a healthy diet, and using prescription medications. Although no signs are visible, the following are common: itching, frequent urination, constancy of thirst, slow healing of bruises and wounds, itching, and a reduction in weight that has no other explanation.

• Paresthesia in the limbs (foot, hands, etc. for example)
Regarding diabetes, what type of treatment is available?
The combination of food, exercise, and medicine is a possible treatment for diabetes, depending on the type and severity of the disease.
You can receive insulin therapy by injections, tablets, or a combination of the two.
There is good news: living a regular and healthy lifestyle is still possible even if you have diabetes. To begin with, you must admit that you have the illness in the first place before you can investigate treatment options.

Given their pivotal role in averting or mitigating the severity of effects associated with sickness, blood sugar monitoring and management are vital. The health problems caused by hyperglycemia, or high blood sugar, include problems with the kidneys, eyes, heart, and blood vessels, to name a few. As well as harm to the kidneys and heart, it can result in blindness and amputation if proper treatment is not received.

If You Have Been Diagnosed With Diabetes, You Must See A Dietitian.

The Reason for Consuming Food:
Even in cases when medication is not being taken to treat diabetes, the most crucial factor in efficient blood sugar management is maintaining a nutritious diet. Regardless of whether you are being treated with insulin injections or pills, you still need to eat well in order to control your diabetes.

In actuality, the so-called "diabetic diet" is a healthy eating regimen that the whole family should adhere to.

A healthy food intake not only helps to regulate blood glucose levels (and therefore avoids the development of diabetic difficulties), but it also helps to maintain body weight and avoid heart disease. Managing blood glucose levels is only one of the many benefits of maintaining a healthy food intake.

Carbohydrates May Be Broken Down Into Two Categories:

- **Foods that are high in carbohydrates**
- **Sweet foods that are available.**

Foods that are high in carbohydrates

Meals that are high in fiber and starch are the ones that are ideal to pick from since they digest slowly and help your body better manage how much glucose is in your blood. Meals that are high in fiber should be consumed more frequently. Some examples of high-fiber foods are high-bran cereals, porridge, brown or wholegrain bread, rice, dried or baked beans, potatoes, roti cooked with brown or wholegrain flour, lentils, oats, and mealie meal, as well as vegetables and fruits with their skins.

• Accompany each meal with a starchy vegetable or grain dish.

• Consuming a meal that contains an excessive amount of carbohydrates (such as potato curry and rice, for example) should be avoided. However, starches do not cause weight gain or make diabetes symptoms worse. This is especially true of starches that are high in fiber.

Meals with a sweet flavor

The body absorbs sugar from sweet meals very fast, which causes blood glucose levels to shoot through the roof. The best alternatives are desserts that are sweetened and have a high percentage of fiber, such as bran muffins. If you absolutely must consume sugary foods, do so in moderation and in conjunction with a meal that is high in fiber rather than as a snack. Consume, for instance, a straightforward cake after a meal rather than as a snack in order to get the most nutrition out of it.

A guide to nibbling on nutritious foods

It's possible that some people need a snack in the middle of the day as well as right before they go to bed. Choose a snack from the list below that is high in fiber:

Exercises for the Management of Diabetes
It is critical to have regular physical activity, which may be accomplished throughout the day by working out three to four times each week for twenty-five to fifty minutes. • Opting to take the stairs rather than the elevator while moving between floors of a building.

• Choosing to walk rather than drive, take a taxi, or get off the bus or taxi a few stops in order to save money on gas.
• Each day, perform between fifty and one hundred skips with a skipping rope.
• Exercises involving the use of weights • Dance
Develop a routine that includes physical activity. Without resorting to the use of medicine, here is how you may successfully reduce your blood sugar levels.

CHAPTER THREE

What Exactly Do Glucose Curves Consist of?

A graph or chart known as the blood glucose curve illustrates how the levels of glucose in the blood fluctuate with time. It shows the changes in blood glucose concentrations that occur during the day. Differences in variables such as meals, physical activity, sleep, or other things often cause these changes.

Your body gets the majority of the glucose it needs from the meals you consume, but it can also produce some glucose on its own. Your cells mostly use glucose for energy. Blood glucose levels can be measured in milligrams per deciliter (mg/dL) or milliliters per liter (mmoL/L). Your body's hormones, including insulin, are responsible for maintaining blood glucose homeostasis, which is measured in either unit.

Numerous different events could have an impact on this process, and some of them could result in significant increases or decreases in glucose levels, which could have long-term effects on one's health. You may be able to obtain a better knowledge of your body's glucose metabolism, find trends, and make informed decisions to promote blood sugar homeostasis by analyzing the glucose curve.

Glucose Curves And Their Appropriate Etiquette

As was said before, glucose metabolism is a complicated process in which the body manages glucose, a kind of sugar that functions as a cell's main source of fuel. The body regulates this sugar. After a meal, glucose from the food enters the circulation, which leads to an increase in the amount of glucose in the blood.

Non-dietary factors, such as mental stress, can also affect your blood glucose levels. In reaction to hyperglycemia, the pancreas releases hormone that controls blood sugar levels, known as insulin. Beta cells in the pancreas produce insulin.

Maintaining normal blood sugar levels involves a number of activities, one of which is insulin's role in facilitating cellular glucose uptake from the circulation for use as an energy source or storage for later.

How exactly does the glucose curve play a role in this scenario? It does this by showing how the levels of glucose in your blood alter in reaction to meals over a period, which highlights how food impacts your body. Your blood glucose levels will typically rise when you eat, and the curve will progressively ascend after that. The rate at which this spike occurs and the degree to which it does so are both determined by a number of different factors, including the kind of food that is consumed and how sensitive you are to insulin.

When blood sugar levels go higher, the pancreas releases insulin; this, in turn, causes blood glucose levels to fall.

After this point, your glucose curve will begin to plummet gradually as the glucose is used by the body or stored. The Significance of Keeping Tabs on Your Blood Glucose Levels

According to the findings of a recent study conducted in the United States, just 12% of Americans have a healthy metabolic profile. If you want to enhance your metabolic health and make healthier choices for your lifestyle, tracking and monitoring your glucose curves may help you do both of those things.

The levels of glucose in your blood may tell you a lot about how your body responds to the many foods,

activities, and lifestyle choices that are part of your typical day. You can identify patterns, trends, and potential triggers that may impact your ability to keep your blood glucose under control if you own a log of your glucose levels over time and follow them.

If you keep your blood glucose levels within 70 to 140 mg/dL for the majority of the day, you may lower your chance of developing conditions like prediabetes or type 2 diabetes.

This information enables you to make educated decisions regarding your food, exercise regimen, stress management, and other lifestyle factors that have a direct influence on your glucose metabolism. As a result, you are able to make choices that are proactive and support your overall health and wellness.

Different Approaches To Interpreting Glucose Curves.

There are a few different approaches to determining the glucose level in the blood. When you interpret the data on your glucose level, whether it comes from a glucometer, a continuous glucose monitor, or a blood sample, you are able to get insights into how your body reacts to a number

of aspects related to your lifestyle and make decisions that are more beneficial to your health.

In Order To Aid You In The Interpretation Of Your Glucose Curves, The Following Guidelines Have Been Provided:

1) Use a CGM to keep track of and monitor your blood glucose levels.

Continuous glucose monitoring (CGM), also known as blood sugar monitoring on a continuous basis, has the potential to revolutionize glucose monitoring and management. Continuous glucose monitors (CGMs) give a more complete and accurate picture of how your body reacts to various diets, activities, and lifestyle choices by providing continuous, real-time data on blood glucose levels.

A CGM is able to monitor your glucose levels throughout the day and provide you with beneficial information that may aid you in making adjustments to your lifestyle that are more conducive to healthy living. Consider enrolling in the CGM program offered by Nutrients if you are interested in getting started with a CGM and learning about the advantages of continuous glucose monitoring.

Nutrients provides you with simple CGM solutions, support from industry professionals, and individualized insights to assist you in making educated decisions and regaining command of your metabolic health.

2) Be aware of spikes in glucose levels and the implications they have

As you may already be aware, an increase in glucose levels may be caused by a variety of causes, one of which is your food. The amount of glucose that is present in the blood after a person has eaten a meal is referred to as postprandial glucose.

Postprandial glucose levels are affected by a number of factors, such as the composition of the meal, the size of the portion, the rate of digestion and absorption, the time of day, and the capacity of the body to manufacture and make use of insulin.

Glucose surges after meals may be an indication of poor regulation of glucose levels and may also raise the risk of illnesses such as diabetes.

3) Research glycemic variability and its connection to overall glucose control.

The swings and changes that occur in a person's blood glucose levels throughout a specific amount of time are referred to as glycemic variability. A condition known as high glycemic variability is characterized by large fluctuations in the amounts of glucose found in the blood, including frequent spikes and decreases.
Better management of blood glucose levels with fewer fluctuations is indicative of low glycemic variability. Suppose you are able to interpret glycemic variability. In that case, you will have a better understanding of the various elements that may be contributing to your feelings of exhaustion, weight gain, inability to sleep, and other metabolic impacts.

4) To get a whole picture, take into account both your fasting and basal glucose levels.

THE GLUCOSE UPSET

Everyone's fasting and basal glucose levels are different, and these differences can be caused by a variety of variables, including age, health conditions, medications used, diet, and lifestyle choices.

Glucose levels during fasting, which are taken first thing in the morning before taking anything to eat or drink, serve as a baseline reference point for the control of

glucose levels. They show the levels of glucose in the body after the subject has abstained from food for at least eight hours.

Some people are of the opinion that there is a connection between fasting glucose levels and resting glucose levels. The capacity of the body to maintain glucose homeostasis may be seen in these numbers when there is no significant impact from the outside World on the levels of glucose in the blood.

The control of your glucose levels may be evaluated using these measures in addition to aspects related to your food and lifestyle. High findings might suggest that you have a predisposition to having metabolic health problems.

Why You May Need More Glucose, Also Known as Carbohydrates

As was said earlier, it is extremely important to have a solid understanding of how your blood sugar levels work and how your body reacts, in particular to the consumption of glucose. Nonetheless, a number of news organizations and sectors of the medical profession have presented glucose as the antagonist in this conflict. When certain conditions are met, it may be helpful to consume

more dietary glucose, commonly referred to as complex carbs, which come from healthy sources.

During all stages of pregnancy, a woman's need for glucose is far higher than what is considered normal in order to provide for the needs of a growing fetus. As a result of this, pregnant women should not reduce the amount of carbohydrates they consume in their diet. Some people, particularly women, find that ingesting a small quantity of carbs before engaging in physical activity enhances both their performance and their overall well-being. This is especially true for marathon runners. If you eat carbs before you work out, your body will use the energy it receives from those carbohydrates immediately rather than storing it.

People who are experiencing a great deal of stress in their lives. Your body has a greater need for glucose in order to function well while you are under a lot of stress. It's possible that increasing the amount of carbs you consume on a daily basis can help you deal with stress better. Those who engage in activities that demand a large amount of mental work should keep in mind that the brain uses about 20% of the glucose that the body needs to

function properly. If you participate in a lot of mental work on a regular basis, you might want additional carbs that are high in nutrients.

The most important thing to take away from this is that not all carbs are unhealthy for you and that different people have different needs in terms of how much they need to consume in order to feel their best. In the course of my therapeutic work, I've observed that this is particularly the case for a subset of female patients who adhere to extremely low-carbohydrate diets (often because they've been led to believe that this is their best course of action). Patients frequently report experiencing a considerable improvement in their symptoms after gradually increasing the amount of carbohydrates in their diet while taking care not to consume an excessive amount of such foods as whole fruit and potatoes.

Management of Blood Sugar and Psychological Well-Being

I'd like to give a quick overview of the correlation between healthy blood sugar levels and mental well-being. Poor control of blood sugar is a key factor that is frequently ignored despite the fact that poor mental health

is a complicated issue with a wide variety of probable causes of the problem. The glucose upset can give rise to feelings of worry, irritability, melancholy, and even a tendency to be more judgmental of oneself and others.

For instance, one study looked at how high glucose levels affected people's ability to make good choices in social situations. Participants may either consume a breakfast that induced a large surge in glucose levels or one that caused a smaller rise in glucose levels. They were then invited to take part in a scenario in which they were given the opportunity to dish out punishment to someone who had committed an offense. Those individuals who reported a greater rise in glucose levels after breakfast were disciplined more severely than those individuals who experienced a lesser increase after breakfast.

According to the theory, the massive rise decreased the amount of tyrosine (a neurotransmitter) in the brain, which caused the individuals' moods to shift more noticeably.
Analyzing your glucose spikes and the balance of your blood sugar, in addition to keeping a record of your

symptoms, may be advantageous if you are struggling with mental health concerns.

Healthy Foods to Eat to Maintain Normal Blood Sugar Levels.

The following foods may be purchased online, in addition to being sold in the majority of supermarkets and health food stores:

• Invest in bread made from whole wheat.

- You should get pumpernickel bread.
- You should go shopping for sweet potatoes. Get yourself some yams at the store.
- You should get some oatmeal at the store.
- You should go shopping for oat bran.
- Go for your nuts shopping.
- You should get some yogurt and garlic.

CONCLUTION

Patients with diabetes sometimes notice rises in their blood sugar levels shortly after eating. The condition of having high blood sugar is referred to as hyperglycemia in the medical field. Insulin, other drugs, or alterations to one's eating routine can frequently be used to bring these spikes under control.

When a person's blood sugar levels continue to rise unchecked, they put themselves at risk for developing issues. There is a possibility that some of these might prove fatal.

People may assist themselves in avoiding issues by adopting a preventative lifestyle that includes a balanced diet and adequate exercise, as well as by working with their doctor to get the optimal diabetic prescription and dose, and by doing both of these things at the same time. People who do not have diabetes might occasionally experience rises in their blood sugar levels. This might be the result of illness, a physical blow, or mental or emotional strain.

Blood sugar can be negatively impacted by not getting enough sleep, feeling stressed out, and drinking too much alcohol. As a consequence of this, treatments pertaining to lifestyle must also be addressed in addition to nutrition. In clinical trials, bebeerine was proven to lower increases in blood sugar by 25% after treatment, and it also has a low risk of adverse effects.

Cinnamon and fenugreek are two spices that do not normally provide any health risks. They may have a beneficial effect on your blood sugar if you consume them in conjunction with a meal that contains carbohydrates.

There is some evidence that chromium and magnesium can help improve insulin sensitivity. There is some evidence to suggest that they could be more successful when they work together.

Vinegar, when consumed alongside carbohydrates, has been found to boost insulin responsiveness and assist in the management of blood sugar levels.

Dehydration has a detrimental impact on the ability to manage blood sugar levels develop an intolerance for insulin, which can cause this disorder, an individual's body may the development of type 2 diabetes.

The digestion of carbohydrates and the release of sugar into the blood can be slowed down by fiber. It has also been shown to suppress appetite and the amount of food consumed.

Regular exercise improves the body's sensitivity to insulin and encourages the removal of blood sugar by cells.

Being obese makes it more difficult for your body to maintain healthy levels of blood sugar. Even a little loss of weight can help in maintaining proper blood sugar levels. The majority of sugar's calories are completely pointless. It induces an increase in blood sugar levels almost immediately, and researchers have linked excessive consumption to insulin resistance.

Refined carbohydrates have a low nutritional value and are linked to weight gain and an increased risk of acquiring type 2 diabetes.

By preventing increases in blood sugar, a diet that is low in carbohydrates might make it easier to lose weight.

Keeping track of your carbohydrates might also be beneficial.

www.ingramcontent.com/pod-product-compliance
Lightning Source LLC
Chambersburg PA
CBHW070743260726
48660CB00007B/2960